A Manual for the

ARTIFICIAL INSEMINATION

OF

QUEEN BEES

BY

OTTO MACKENSEN and **W. C. ROBERTS**

Division of Bee Culture

United States Department of Agriculture

Agricultural Research Administration

Bureau of Entomology and Plant Quarantine

A Manual for the Artificial Insemination of Queen Bees
© Otto Mackensen and W. C. Roberts

This is a reprint by Northern Bee Books of the manual originally published by P. W. Stanley, F.R.E.S. of Badgerdell Apiaries UK by courtesy of the U.S. Department of Agriculture

ISBN 978-1-908904-27-0

Published by Northern Bee Books, 2013
Scout Bottom Farm
Mytholmroyd
Hebden Bridge
HX7 5JS (UK)

Design and artwork
D&P Design and Print
Worcestershire

Printed by Lightning Source, UK

A Manual for the

ARTIFICIAL INSEMINATION

OF

QUEEN BEES

BY

OTTO MACKENSEN and **W. C. ROBERTS**

CONTENTS

ILLUSTRATIONS

A MANUAL FOR

THE ARTIFICIAL INSEMINATION OF QUEEN BEES

By OTTO MACKENSEN and W. C. ROBERTS*

(Division of Bee Culture)

INTRODUCTION

Ever since the discovery that the queen mates in the air, the control of mating has been the bee breeder's dream. A number of methods have been devised for controlling the natural mating act, of which isolation at mating stations has been the most satisfactory. It has long been realized, however, that absolute control of mating could only be attained through some method of artificial insemination, and many efforts have been made in this direction with varying degrees of success.

The many early attempts at artificial insemination have been reviewed by Nolan (5) and, although the early investigators have advanced the method, the works which have contributed most are those of Watson (9, 10), Nolan (5, 6), and Laidlaw (2). By modifying the apparatus and methods devised by these three men, the writers have been able to obtain results far superior to any heretofore presented, and it is the purpose of this publication to describe the apparatus and procedure in sufficient detail so that anyone may duplicate them.†

THE REPRODUCTIVE ORGANS

To be successful with artificial insemination one must be familiar with certain anatomical features of the queen. Although several workers have studied the sex organs of bees, Laidlaw (2) made the most recent and thorough study from an artificial insemination standpoint, and was the first to recognize the full significance of the valvefold of the queen in the success of the insemination process.

The tip of the abdomen of the queen is made up of an upper (or dorsal) plate, and a lower (or ventral) plate, which close at the tip like a clam shell. The cavity that these plates enclose is called the sting chamber. In figure 1 the tip of the abdomen is shown in proper position for artificial insemination, with the dorsal plate (DP) and the ventral plate (VP) drawn apart, exposing the sting chamber and its various structures, including the sting (ST) and the vaginal orifice (VO).

* In co-operation with the Louisiana State University and the University of Wisconsin.

† The insemination apparatus, exclusive of microscope and anesthetic equipment, can be purchased from the Department of Economic Entomology, King Hall, University of Wisconsin, Madison, Wis.

Figure 2 illustrates the internal portions of the reproductive tract with the side toward the observer removed. The dorsal and ventral plates and the sting are not shown, but portions of the walls of the sting chamber are seen at the right. A fold across the anterior floor of the sting chamber loosely separates a region called the bursa copulatrix from the sting chamber proper. The Vagina (V), through its vaginal orifice (VO), and the bursal pouches (BP) open into this region. There are two bursal pouches, their openings lying at the side of and below the vaginal orifice. Only the left pouch is shown in figure 2. The position of their openings in relation to the vagina, when the queen is properly mounted for insemination, is shown in figure 1, BP. They are easily found with a dull probe. Sometimes, when the queen is poorly mounted, a beginner might mistake a bursal pouch for the vagina.

The spermathecal duct (SPD) from the spermatheca (not shown) enters the vagina anteriorly from above. Just below the opening of this duct is the valvefold (VF), a large tonguelike structure with transverse ridges, which makes it distinguishable from other tissues when viewed through the vaginal opening. Its position is such that it can close the passage between the vagina and the median oviduct (SH and K) with a valvelike action. The paired oviducts (POV) enter the median oviduct anteriorly. Each paired oviduct leads to an ovary (not shown). They are large fluted structures capable of great expansion for the temporary storage of sperm after mating and of eggs in a laying queen. In figure 2 the reproductive tract is extended. During insemination the queen is held in such a way that the vagina is collapsed, and the valvefold often appears to lie just inside the vaginal opening (fig. 1, VF).

Laidlaw found the diameter of the vaginal orifice to vary from 0.65 to 0.68 mm., and the average diameter of the oviduct orifice to be 0.33 mm. These diameters are important considerations in syringe construction.

A detailed knowledge of the anatomy of the drone reproductive organs is not necessary for the mastery of the insemination technique. A description of their structure and function is given by Laidlaw (2). During natural mating the penis everts, and the reproductive fluids are ejaculated probably more or less simultaneously with the eversion. The semen, a cream-colored fluid containing the sperm, passes out first and is followed by the mucus, which is more viscous, pure white, and coagulates after ejaculation. Further details about the ejaculation process are given under Insemination Procedure.

Queens just returned from the mating flight have been studied by a number of investigators. According to Laidlaw (2), who reviewed the earlier work, most of the semen is found in the oviducts, some is in the vagina, and some has already migrated into the spermathecal duct and spermatheca. Parts of the penis are found in the sting chamber buried in mucus, which also extends into the folds of its walls.

Since the penis apparently does not enter the vagina, the queen probably lowers the valvefold during the mating act to permit the semen to pass.

In order to get the semen in its natural position by artificial insemination, the valvefold must be pushed ventrally to permit the point of the syringe to pass into the median oviduct. If the syringe enters only the mouth of the vagina, the semen presses the valvefold against the median oviduct and is forced back around the syringe and out into the sting chamber. The vagina is not easily distendable, but the oviducts expand to take care of a large quantity of semen.

EQUIPMENT AND CONSTRUCTION OF INSTRUMENTS
Microscope and Light

The major equipment needed to perform the artificial insemination operation is illustrated in figure 3, and the manipulating apparatus with instruments in place is shown in more detail from the side of the operator in figure 4. The binocular dissecting microscope should preferably be one provided with a revolving nosepiece or other mechanism making adjustment from low to high power easy. The low power should give a magnification of about 6 diameters, and the high power about 20 diameters. A single intermediate magnification can be used. When two powers are used, sperm is taken into the syringe under low power and injected under high power. A still higher magnification will be found useful in making and measuring instruments. An attached lamp that always illuminates the focal point of the microscope is a great convenience.

Carbon Dioxide Equipment

Carbon dioxide serves as an anesthetic. The equipment for its application is illustrated in figure 3. This gas is obtained in cylinders from wholesale grocers or similar supply houses. To reduce the high pressure in the cylinder, a regulator is provided which permits adjustment to a delivery pressure of 4 to 5 pounds per square inch. A needle valve permits adjustment of the flow of gas to a very fine stream. A rubber tube carries the gas to the queen holder by way of a three-way stopcock, which permits diversion of the stream of gas while the queen is being mounted, without disturbing the needle-valve adjustment. Another line leads into a jar, in which queens are given additional anesthetizations to be described later.

The Manipulating Apparatus

The manipulating apparatus is a stand (fig. 4) on which the queen holder (QH), the syringe (S), and holding hooks (VH and STH) are mounted in such a way that they can be adjusted or manipulated. It is essentially the same as the apparatus developed by Nolan (5), with modifications which make more accurate adjustment possible. The stage (ST) is made of a piece of $\frac{1}{4}$-inch iron plate, 3 inches wide and 11 inches long, raised at each end by a piece of wood thick enough to permit the microscope base to slip under the stage. The weight of the stage gives stability to the apparatus. Two upright $\frac{3}{8}$-inch brass rods threaded at the bottom end are screwed into the stage at the points illustrated, and to these rods all other parts are attached. The rod at the left of the operator is 3 inches high and the one to the right $3\frac{1}{2}$ inches. These rods are $4\frac{1}{2}$ inches apart center to center.

The mount for the queen holder is made of wood, and consists of a queen-holder mounting block (QHMB) attached to a horizontal strip (HS). The strip is $\frac{1}{2}$ by $\frac{3}{4}$ by 6 inches, with a hole bored near each end so that it can slip up and down on the two posts and with set screws to hold it fast at any desired level. Near the right-hand post is a horizontal slot about 2 inches long. A long bolt passing through this slot and also through the block makes it possible to adjust the block at any desired angle. The queen holder (QH) fits into a hole in this block, and a set screw holds it securely in place. A wide groove is cut on the set-screw side of the hole, and a piece of leather tacked to the top of the block fits into this groove preventing the set screw from scratching or breaking the queen holder. It also keeps the queen holder in place by light friction until the set screw can be tightened. The set screw works in a hole bored just small enough for the threads to take hold.

Since the mountings for the syringe (S), the ventral hook (VH), and the sting hook (STH) are essentially similar, a detailed description of the syringe mounting will suffice for all three. A block of wood, the syringe mounting block (SMB), is bored so that it will fit snugly over the post as illustrated. On the left side of the post this block is divided by a vertical saw cut, and a $\frac{3}{16}$-inch bolt is provided with which the separated parts can be pulled together if necessary to increase friction on the post. This bolt may have a wing nut, or one side of the divided block may be bored to a smaller diameter. In any case the head of the bolt must be flat enough not to interfere with the movement of the syringe.

On the other side of the post the syringe holder (SH) is attached to the block. The syringe holder is simply a piece of sheet metal cut and bent into the shape of a box $\frac{1}{2}$ by $\frac{1}{2}$ by $1\frac{1}{2}$ inches. The $\frac{1}{8}$ by 1 inch bolt $\frac{1}{2}$ inch from one end holds the bottom of this box to the block. This bolt projects about $\frac{1}{2}$ inch back of the block, and a piece of coil spring is put on under the nut so that the friction between the box and the block can be increased or decreased by tightening or loosening the nut. In each end of the box a hole is bored of such a size that the syringe will slip through easily but not loosely. A curved piece of clock mainspring (SP) slipped in between the syringe and the side of the box holds the syringe in place. The curvature of this spring can be adjusted to permit the syringe to slip in and out easily but still stay in place when released. The ventral hook and sting hook are mounted in the same way, except that the boxes for them are $\frac{3}{8}$ by $\frac{3}{8}$ by $1\frac{1}{2}$ inches.

It is important to keep the syringe and the hook handles clean and polished with oil or a hard wax to make them slip easily. If the wooden parts are treated with wax, they will not expand and contract excessively with changes in humidity.

Queen Holder

The queen holder (fig. 5) is a modification of the type devised by Jas. I. Hambleton and first used extensively by Nolan (5). It is a tube slightly constricted at one end, into which a long stopper fits snugly. The queen is made to back into the holder until her abdomen protrudes from the small end and then is held in place by the stopper. Both parts are made of Lucite, a transparent plastic. The stopper is also a tube, which permits a stream of carbon dioxide to flow gently over the queen, keeping her anesthetized during the insemination operation. The drilling and polishing of Lucite are discussed later under Plastic Syringe.

Dimensions are given of the holder used successfully by the authors. There can be some flexibility of dimensions, but it is well to remember that the thoraxes of most well-developed queens range in diameter from 0.195 to 0.205 inch. The opening at the end of the holder may be from 0.18 to 0.19 inch in diameter. The $\frac{7}{8}$-inch taper is adequate to permit only the last three segments of the queen to protrude from the holder. This taper may be obtained by stretching the plastic tube after heating, as described under construction of the syringe tip, or by drilling with a succession of drills. Several small grooves should be cut with a three-cornered file on the inside of the holder at the tapered end to facilitate the escape of gas.

The stopper diameter must be very near the diameter of the holder (0.257 inch) to move in and out of the holder with sufficient friction to remain firm at any place. If the stopper loses friction through wear, its diameter may be increased with a light coat of plastic cement or lacquer. The slight protuberance at the front end of the stopper has four additional lateral outlets (not shown in diagram). This protuberance aids in adjusting the queen in the holder and protects her antennae from being mashed. The enlarged knob at the posterior end holds the rubber tubing onto the stopper. The stream of carbon dioxide from the cylinder passes through the stopper, is dispersed by the five openings at the end of the stopper, and flows over the queen and out the end of the holder.

If facilities are not available for making the plastic queen holder, a glass one is easily made by drawing 9-mm. glass tubing to about 4 mm. outside diameter, finding the right inside diameter for the small end, breaking at this point, and grinding off the edges. Since commercial glass tubing varies in size, it is necessary to select a piece of the proper inside diameter from the 9-mm. size.

The stopper is a piece of spongy paper, such as paper toweling, rolled over a match stick, which is later pushed out to make a thick-walled tube. If the tube is of the right size, friction with the walls of the glass holder keeps it in place. It is made long enough to project from the glass holder when the queen is in place, and additional paper is glued onto this end to make it taper. If preferred, the carbon dioxide supply tube can easily be slipped on and off the tapered end at each operation, and the three-way stopcock eliminated.

Syringe

The syringe is a modification of the instruments used by other workers in this field. It consists of a small tube inside of which a tightly fitting plunger draws in and expels the semen. Two types of syringes are being used.

Glass Syringe. For the glass syringe, a glass tube is employed as a plunger barrel. This tube will hereafter be referred to as the glass tip or simply the tip. A brass spring wire serves as a plunger, and a mechanical pencil, as recommended by Nolan (6), provides the mechanism for moving the plunger. The glass tip is attached to the end of the pencil housing, and the plunger takes the place of the lead. A number of special tools and materials are needed for a construction of this type.

For drawing capillary glass tubing an ordinary bunsen burner will do, but a blast burner is a great convenience where both gas and air are available. A gasoline blow-torch has been found very satisfactory.

A jewelers' fine-grain glass-grinding wheel is needed for grinding off glass tips to the right diameter. Such a wheel can easily be mounted on a shaft and made to turn slowly by means of a belt and motor. The lower part of the wheel should dip into a tray of water to keep it flooded as it turns. The cooling action of the water prevents chipping of the glass.

A special gas burner is needed for producing a fine flame for use in forming the tapered end of the glass tips. This burner can be a piece of 6-mm. glass tubing drawn to an inside diameter of 0.3 mm. at one end. The burner is attached to an ordinary gas outlet, which is adjusted to produce a flame about 3 mm. in diameter.

A compound microscope equipped with a micrometer eyepiece and having a magnification of about 60 diameters is useful in measuring the diameter of the glass tips as well as other small parts of the insemination equipment while under construction. Some of these measurements can be made with an ordinary micrometer. If a compound microscope is not available, a micrometer eyepiece can be used in the dissecting microscope with a magnification of about 60 diameters.

A number of small tools that can be obtained from jewelers' supply houses are needed. They include No. 6 cut files of various shapes, small flat-nose and pointed-nose pliers, and rods and triangular slips of fine-grain Arkansas stone. The end of a rod is ground on a coarser stone to a cone-shaped tip, which is used in grinding the inside edges of the capillary tubing. These tools are also used in making the holding hooks and vaginal probe.

A supply of No. 26 B. and S. gage wire should be on hand for making plungers. Several kinds of wire will do, but spring brass is preferred because it is stiff, yet solders well, and does not corrode easily.

6

Some mechanical pencils are better adapted for syringe making than others. One having a round housing and using a 4-inch lead has been found most satisfactory. This type has a stationary, hollow metal core with a slot running its entire length. The lead and lead holder slide in this core, and a spiral made of steel wire or a steel strip encloses almost its entire length. Projections on the lead holder extend through the slot into the spiral, and as the spiral is turned the holder slides, moving the lead in or out of the pencil.

A number of changes must be made to adapt a pencil to its new use. The friction that keeps the lead at the adjusted level must be eliminated. Usually the pencil must be taken apart to accomplish this. Since the friction is caused in different ways in different makes of pencils, the exact procedure cannot be described. The point of the pencil is sawed or filed off sufficiently to let the lead holder project. If the housing is hexagonal, it should be replaced with a round tube, preferably of solderable material. The lead holder should be filed to a smaller diameter to allow more play between it and the core, or it can be replaced entirely with a piece of wire bent and filed into shape. When the pencil is reassembled the spiral should turn without friction.

For the plunger a piece of 26 B. and S. gage brass spring wire is selected which has no kinks to prevent a tight fit. Any gentle bend resulting from the wire being wound on a spool may be straightened by pulling the wire between thumb and forefinger a number of times, but sharp kinks are difficult to remove and should be avoided. One end of the wire is ground off squarely, and the burred edges are polished. Then after the wire has been cut to the proper length, the other end is soldered into the hollow end of the lead holder. The length of the plunger will depend upon the construction of the pencil and on the length of the completed glass tip. It should be slightly longer than the tip, and long enough not to slip out of its upper end when withdrawn as far into the pencil as possible. If there is still some bend in the plunger, it should be attached so that the back of the arch will rub against one of the sides of the core. Such a position will prevent the arch from pushing the end of the glass tip against the spiral and possibly breaking it, and at the same time will prevent the end of the plunger from slipping out of the core groove when drawn into the pencil while no glass tip is present.

To make a good glass tip requires some practice and the exercise of proper care. The first step is to draw out a supply of capillary tubing. Ordinary 6-mm. soft-glass tubing has been found very satisfactory for this purpose. Long sections of fairly uniform bore can best be obtained by heating a section of tubing about 1 inch long, drawing slowly at first until the center of the section is of about the right diameter, and then drawing more rapidly to a length of 3 to 4 feet. With 26 gage (0.41-mm.) wire the inside diameter is tested until a piece of nearly uniform bore about 60 mm. long is found which fits closely. The glass is broken at the point where the end of the wire fitted most tightly, and this end is made the inside end; the larger end becomes the point of the syringe. The inner edge of the small end is ground under water by twirling on the pointed Arkansas stone, so that there will be no sharp edge to scratch the plunger and gradually decrease its diameter. The plunger should not be inserted from this end until the glass tip is completed and ready for mounting, and then only under the microscope, because the glass is easily broken if the plunger is not inserted perfectly straight.

The large end of the tip is drawn to a smaller diameter to form the point of the syringe. To do this heat a spot near the end in the small gas flame and draw the ends to a diameter of somewhat less than 0.27 mm. Sometimes two or three attempts must be made before a satisfactory product is obtained. The drawn section is then scratched with the sharp edge of a stone, broken off at the proper point, and ground back to an outside diameter of 0.27 mm. The outside edge is ground off lightly on the grinding wheel and the inside edge by spinning between thumb and forefinger on the pointed stone under water, or with a drop of water covering the point. The point is then polished until it appears perfectly smooth when magnified about 60 times, by twirling the tip on the end of a soft piece of wood rubbed with jewelers' rouge, or by holding it against such a piece of wood mounted on the end of a motor shaft. The completed tip should be 35 to 50 mm. long. To attach it to the pencil, put it over the plunger and draw it into the pencil until it sticks out about 25 mm., then glue it into place with an acetone-soluble cement such as is used to build model airplanes. This cement is easily dissolved when it becomes necessary to replace the tip.

The proper diameters at the point of the glass tip are of utmost importance. The outside diameter must be small enough to permit passage into the oviduct, and yet the inside diameter must be large enough to permit semen to be taken up easily and quickly. The outside diameter should not be over 0.3 mm., and 0.27 mm. is usually satisfactory. The inside diameter should not be less than 0.15 mm. These limits differ slightly from the dimensions recommended for the plastic syringe.

When made as described with 26-gage wire (0.41 mm.), the glass tip has a capacity of 1 mm.^{3} for every 7.6 mm. of length. If a 27-gage (0.36 mm.) plunger is used, the capacity is 1 mm.^{3} for every 9.8 mm. of length. Good instruments have been made with both sizes. Tips of smaller diameter are too delicate and have too small a capacity to be practical. Larger ones are more difficult to finish at the point with a large enough inside diameter and a small enough outside diameter.

Plastic Syringe. The plastic syringe is made of Lucite and brass. Most of its parts must be made on a lathe. The Lucite tip is superior to glass because it is not easily broken, sharp edges are eliminated, and it can be machined and drawn to the desired diameter and bore. Threaded replaceable tips can be readily changed and are easily cleaned. Lucite does not have the surface hardness of glass, and consequently will wear slowly. It softens when heated. Grease and oil can be removed with hexane, naphtha, methanol, or mild soap and water.

The machining qualities of Lucite and brass are similar. Since this plastic is a poor conductor of heat, it is necessary to prevent overheating when drilling, cutting, or polishing. Drills should be lubricated with mineral oil or an oil solution (2 per cent of soluble oil in water). Frequent removal of chips is necessary when deep holes are drilled, and the holes are filled with the oil solution at each removal of the drill. Sharp drills and proper lubrication give uniform and polished inside walls to the tip, which result in good suction without a lubricant.

All the syringe parts are shown in figure 6, and the structural details of the tips and plunger are given in figure 7. Since the measurements and details of construction of the housing, turning screw, couplings, and supplemental rod are of secondary importance, they will not be described. Their approximate size can be ascertained from the picture. The universal joint between the turning screw and the supplemental rod allows the metal plunger to move within the tip without rotating. Lack of rotation reduces wear and gives better suction.

The tip is made from a Lucite rod of 0.1875-inch diameter. This rod is placed in the machine and drilled to a depth of about 1 inch with a No. 72 (0.025 inch) drill. A smaller drill—No. 79 (0.0145 inch)—provided with a long shank is then used to drill an additional 0.1 inch in the bottom of the 0.025-inch hole. The outside diameter is then turned down to 0.164 inch, and the end threaded for a distance of about 0.25 inch with an 8–32 threading die. Before the rod is removed from the machine, its diameter between the threaded portion and the end of the drilled portion can be reduced to the approximate size of the main portion of the tip (0.085 inch).

The end of the tip containing the small hole is then rotated on an electric soldering iron until it becomes soft enough to stretch. This 0.1-inch section with the 0.0145-inch bore is then stretched to a length of 0.2 to 0.25 inch and, while still held taut, is hardened in cold water. If the rod is properly heated, the 0.025-inch hole is not distorted. The 0.0145-inch hole becomes a gradual taper from that diameter down to less than 0.008 inch. The end of the tip is then filed off square, and the outside diameter reduced to 0.012 inch. No. 2 cut files can be used to reduce the diameter to near size, but the polishing should be done with 9/0 production finishing paper. The final polish may be obtained by rubbing with moistened cigar ash.

The plunger can be made from brass spring wire of 0.025-inch diameter. It must be straight and uniformly round without sharp edges. The butt end is soldered into a 0.0625-inch brass rod which has been threaded to screw into the supplemental rod of the syringe.

Holding Hooks

The function of the holding hooks is to hold the sting chamber open and the sting back out of the way during the operation. The ventral hook (figs. 1 and 4, VH; fig. 8) fits over the ventral plate. It is constructed of a piece of No. 24 gage brass wire slightly flattened at the end, and bent as illustrated in figure 8. The distance from the bottom of the U to the tip is 2.5 mm., and the distance between the inside walls of the U is 0.37 mm. The tip of the ventral plate fits into the U-shaped portion so that the plate remains in a vertical position as it is pulled ventrally by the hook.

The dorsal or sting hook (figs. 1 and 4, STH; fig. 8) is designed to pull the entire sting mechanism dorsally. A similar instrument was used by Laidlaw (2). It has an enlargement at the end, which fits into the triangular area between the basal portions of the sting lancets, and extends underneath them (fig. 1). Figure 8 gives a side view of his instrument at A and a top view at B from the angle indicated by the arrow in A. The enlarged tip is 0.77 mm. wide. The thinnest part of the stem is 0.08 mm. when viewed from above and 0.17 mm. when viewed from the side. The stem is bent to fit the queen parts. This instrument is made from wire about 0.92 mm. in diameter, and filed down to the proper shape with jewelers' files. The enlarged tip represents the end of the wire filed off at an angle.

All rough edges of both the ventral and sting hook are polished first with a fine stone and then with jewelers' rouge. Both hooks are soldered to the ends of brass rods $\frac{1}{16}$ inch in diameter and 5 inches long, which serve as handles and fit into the sheet-metal boxes.

Other Equipment

Other items of equipment needed for the operation are a pair of forceps, a sting depressor, a dish of water for cleaning the syringe, a vaginal probe, and a container for treating drones with chloroform.

The sting depressor is simply a dull-pointed dissecting needle.

The probe (fig. 8) is an instrument used to push the valvefold downward. It is a piece of No. 24 gage brass wire bent at right angles 4 mm. from one end. This end is flattened to a thickness of 0.13 mm. on a plane with the main stem of the instrument and polished down to a width of about 0.19 mm. The probe is bent slightly near the tip, so that the main part of the wire does not obstruct the view when the tip is inserted into the vagina.

Drones are made to ejaculate in a 1-by-4-inch glass vial containing paper soaked in chloroform wadded in the bottom. A stopper fastened to the table so that the vial can be put onto it in a horizontal position is a great time saver.

INSEMINATION PROCEDURE

Adjusting the Flow of Carbon Dioxide

The end of the carbon dioxide supply tube is immersed in water and the flow of gas adjusted to a slow bubbling. It should not be faster than is necessary to keep the queen completely anesthetized. Experience will soon show just how much this should be. The tube is then passed through the queenholder mounting block from below, the stopper attached, and the three-way stopcock in the supply line turned, to prevent gas from passing through the stopper while the queen is being mounted.

Preparing the Syringe

To function properly the tip of the glass syringe must be filled with water, which acts as a lubricant and increases the suction of the plunger. Water is first drawn into the tip by withdrawing the plunger. Then, while a finger is held against the end, the plunger is pushed out again until the air around it has been entirely replaced by water. A 5-mm. column of water is left at the end of the plunger.

The plastic syringe can be prepared in much the same way as the glass syringe when a lubricant seems necessary. Ordinarily the water will be present after the rinsing operation described later. The plunger should be pushed out as far as it will go.

Tap water has been found satisfactory, but in some localities distilled water may be better. Physiological salt solution must not be used with the glass syringe. because it cannot be thoroughly rinsed and, when the water dries up, the salt residue freezes the plunger in the tip and corrodes the syringe parts.

Preparing the Queen

The queen is made to walk into a tube similar in size and construction to the queen holder. When she reaches the partly closed end she begins backing up, and if the queen holder is quickly put in place she usually backs into it. The stopper is pushed in after her until her abdomen protrudes from the small end of the holder and she cannot move about readily. For best results, only about the last three segments of the abdomen should protrude.

The three-way stopcock is turned so that carbon dioxide will flow through the queen holder. The queen breathes heavily for a few minutes and then gradually becomes quiet. If her abdomen expands abnormally, the gas is being forced into her abdominal air sacs, an indication that the flow is too strong. Unless very severe this action seems to do no harm, although it makes insemination difficult. The holder is withdrawn into its mounting block by pulling on the carbon dioxide supply tube, and tightened in place by the set screw. The dorsal part of the queen should be at the right of the operator. The queen holder should be about 30° from vertical, with the upper end leaning to the right (fig. 4).

The queen is usually quiet by the time she is completely mounted, and the holding hooks can be put in place. This is done under low-power magnification. First one hook and then the other is inserted into the sting chamber, and the abdominal plates are pulled apart. With the left hand the sting depressor is used to hold the sting down while the sting hook is placed in the triangular area between the bases of the sting lancets, and the sting hook is left in this position to prevent unnecessary drying of the delicate tissues while the syringe is being loaded.

Filling the Syringe

The microscope is withdrawn slightly and the syringe placed in its box, with care not to break the tip. This is done with greatest safety by depressing the spring with forceps while the syringe is being inserted. The microscope and syringe are then so adjusted that the end of the syringe is in focus.

A drone is anesthetized by dropping him in the vial already described. His abdomen contracts and usually the penis partially everts, as illustrated in figure 9, A. He is then made to evert more completely by being squeezed between thumb and forefinger. There is great variation in the degree of eversion, the distribution of semen and mucus, and the amount of semen ejaculated. Eversion usually stops at the stage illustrated in figure 9, B; which is about two-thirds complete. As the process of eversion proceeds, the cream-colored semen passes out first followed by the thicker white mucus. If the eversion process can be stopped at just the right point, a drop of pure semen will be found at the tip with all the mucus left inside. When this ideal situation exists it is very easy to take up the semen. Usually, however, at least some of the mucus comes out after the semen, and the two are distributed on the penis in various arrangements. Often the semen is spread so thinly over the mucus that it is difficult to take up.

It is best to see that an ample supply of drones is available and to use only those that evert and ejaculate most satisfactorily. This is especially important when individual matings are being made, so that the maximum amount of semen is obtained from the single drone used. Movement of sperm causes the semen to spread in a thin layer over the mucus and to mix with it until too thick to be taken into the syringe easily. This mixing also takes place while the drone is partially everted. It is, therefore, important that drones be utilized as soon as possible after anesthetization. Without abdominal contraction semen is rarely obtainable, but when the abdomen contracts without partial eversion the eversion can often be completed by pressure, and a good amount of semen obtained.

The ejaculated drone is brought near the tip of the syringe with the left hand and the plunger withdrawn slightly to make an air bubble. The surface of the semen is then made to touch the point of the syringe at about a 45° angle. If the syringe is raised slightly after contact has been made, the semen will adhere to it and flow toward it as the plunger is withdrawn. This procedure helps to avoid the mucus,

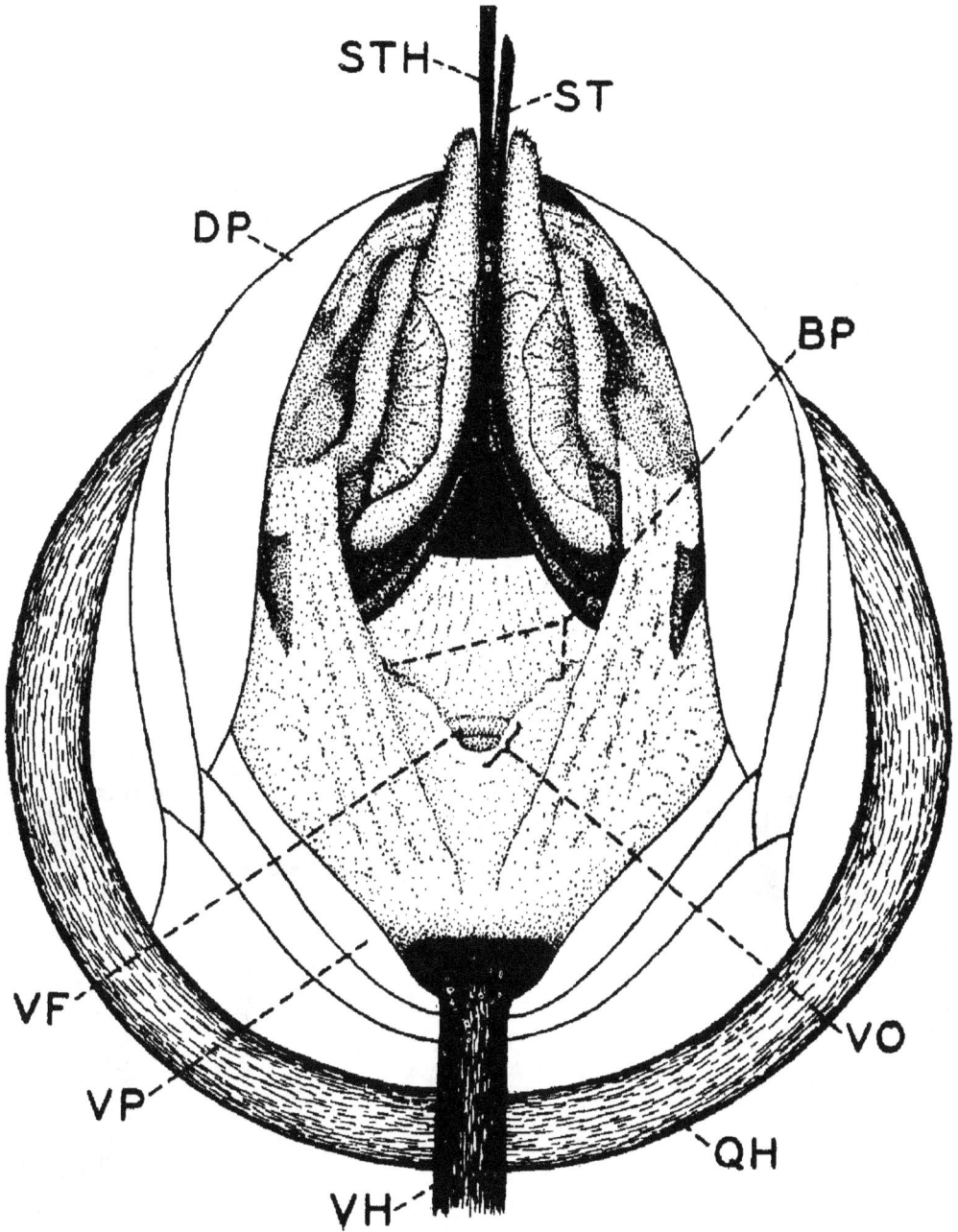

Figure 1.—View of sting chamber of queen properly opened for insemination: BP—Opening of bursal pouches; DP—dorsal plate; QH—queen holder; ST—sting; STH—sting hook; VF—valvefold; VH—ventral hook; VO—vaginal orifice; VP—ventral plate.

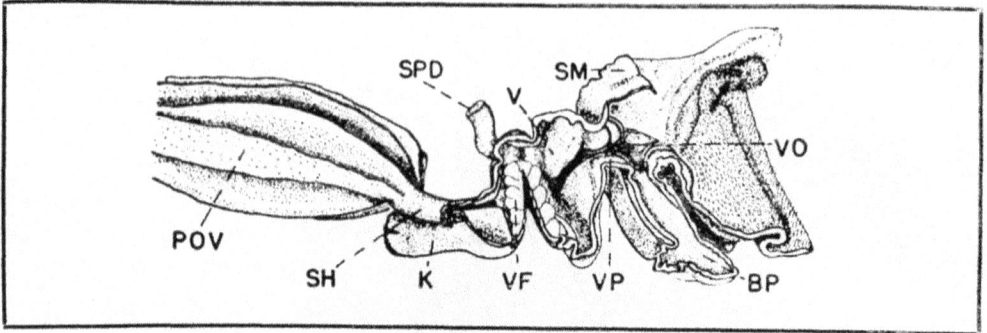

Figure 2.—Reproductive tract of queen caudad of the ovaries, extended, with side removed to show relation of valvefold to median oviduct and vagina: BP—bursal pouch; K—keel of median oviduct; POV—paired oviduct; SH—shelf of median oviduct; SM—sting membrane; SPD—spermathecal duct; V—vagina; VF—valvefold; VO—vaginal orifice; VP—vaginal passage. (From Laidlaw).

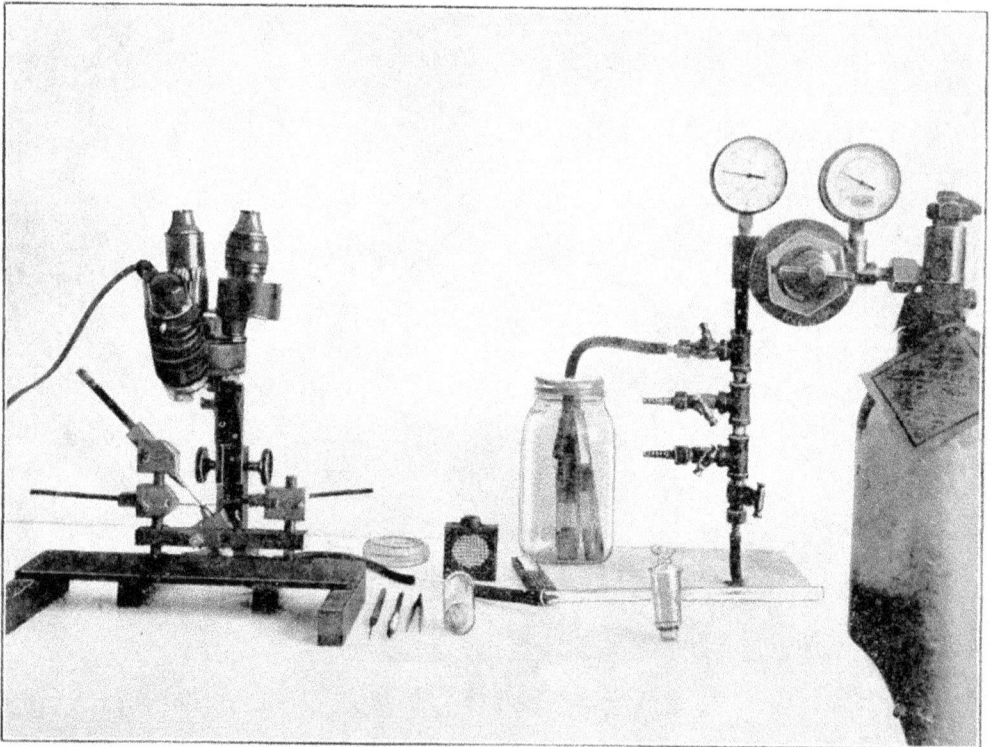

Figure 3.—Complete insemination equipment, showing manipulating apparatus under microscope with queen in place ready for injection of semen, jar for giving additional carbon dioxide treatments, and carbon dioxide cylinder with pressure regulator attached.

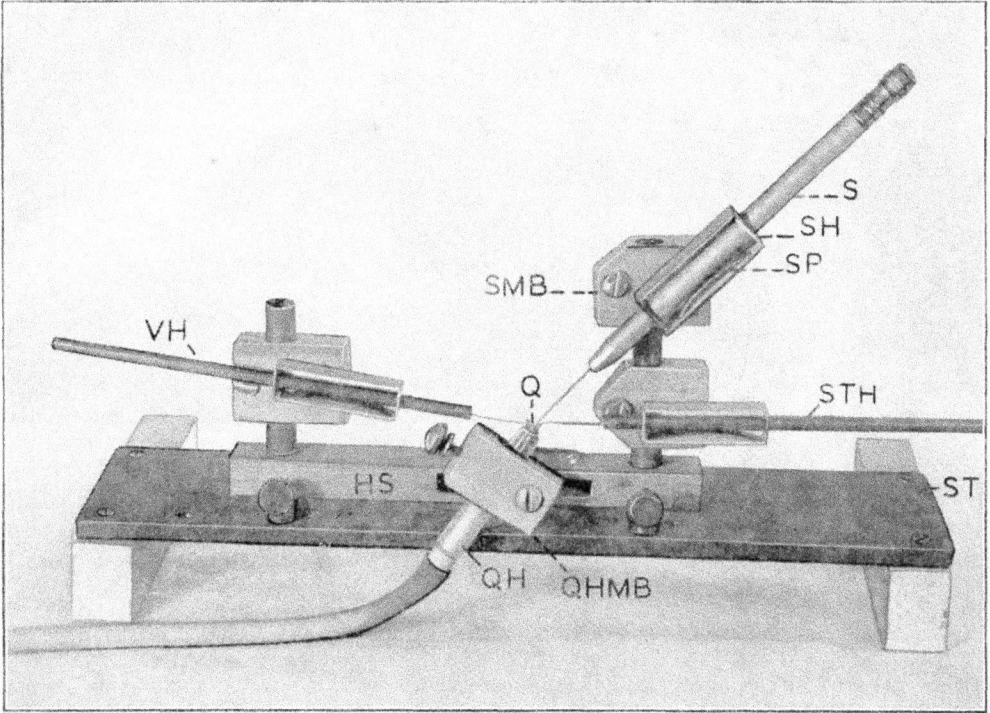

Figure 4.—Manipulating apparatus viewed from operator's side, showing mounting of queen holder, syringe, and holding hooks: **HS**—horizontal strip; **Q**—queen; **QH**—queen holder; **QHMB**—queen holder mounting block; **S**—syringe; **SH**—syringe holder; **SMB**—syringe mounting block; **SP**—spring; **ST**—stage; **STH**—sting hook; **VH**—ventral hook.

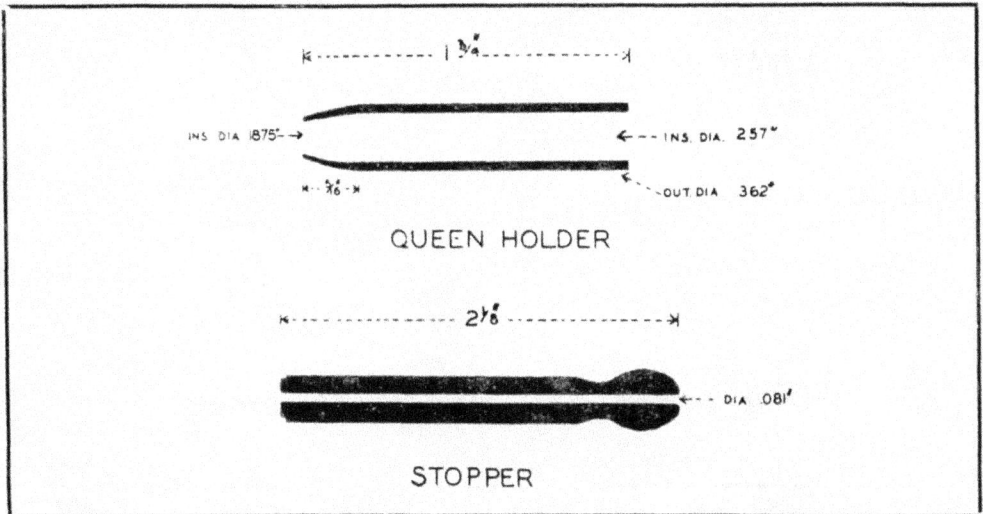

Figure 5.—Structural details of the queen holder.

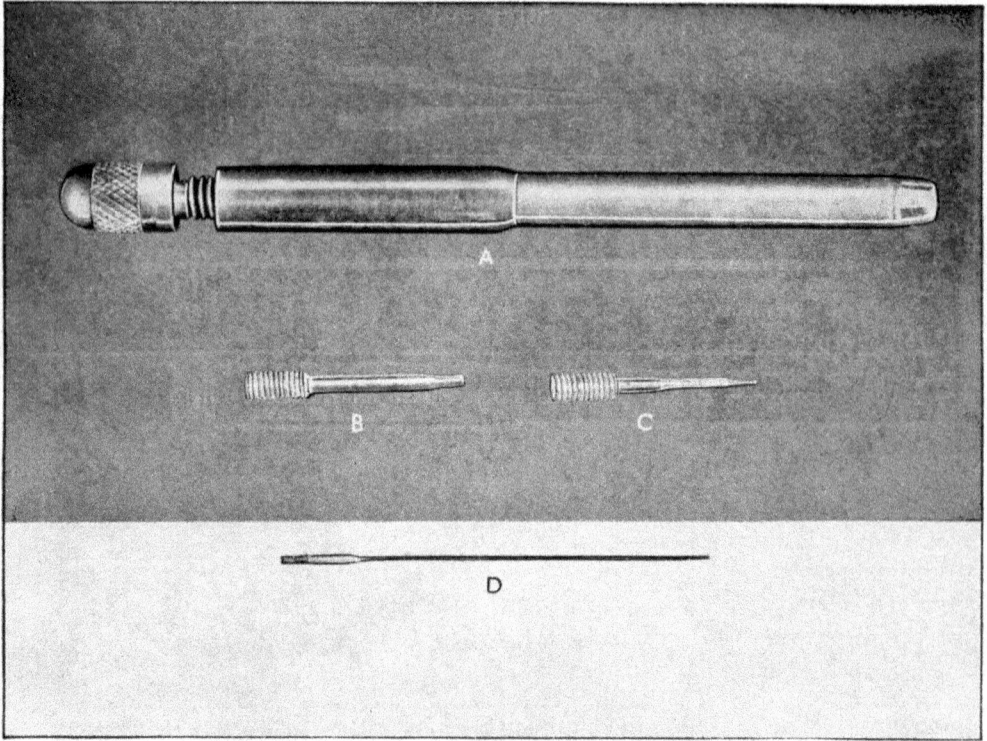

Figure 6.—Parts of syringe: A—turning screw in housing; B—partly finished Lucite tip; C—finished Lucite tip; D—plunger.

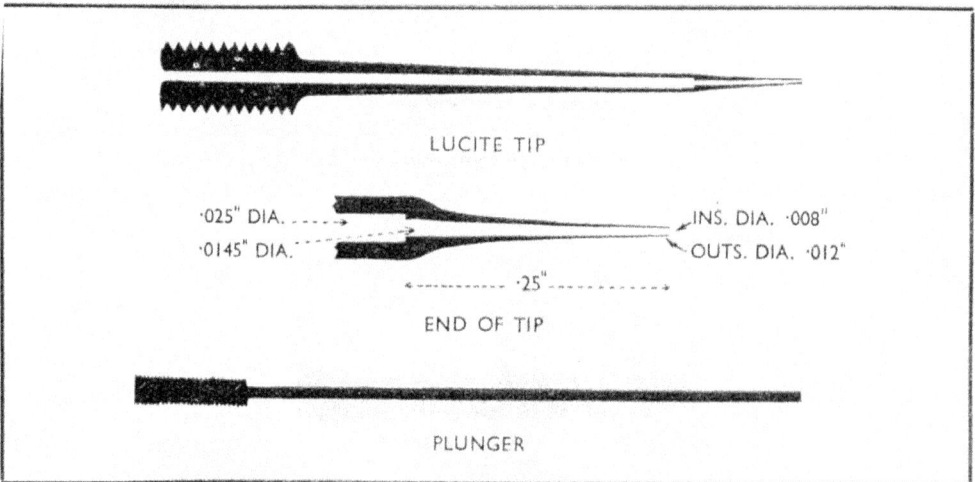

Figure 7.—Structural details of the Lucite tip and its plunger.

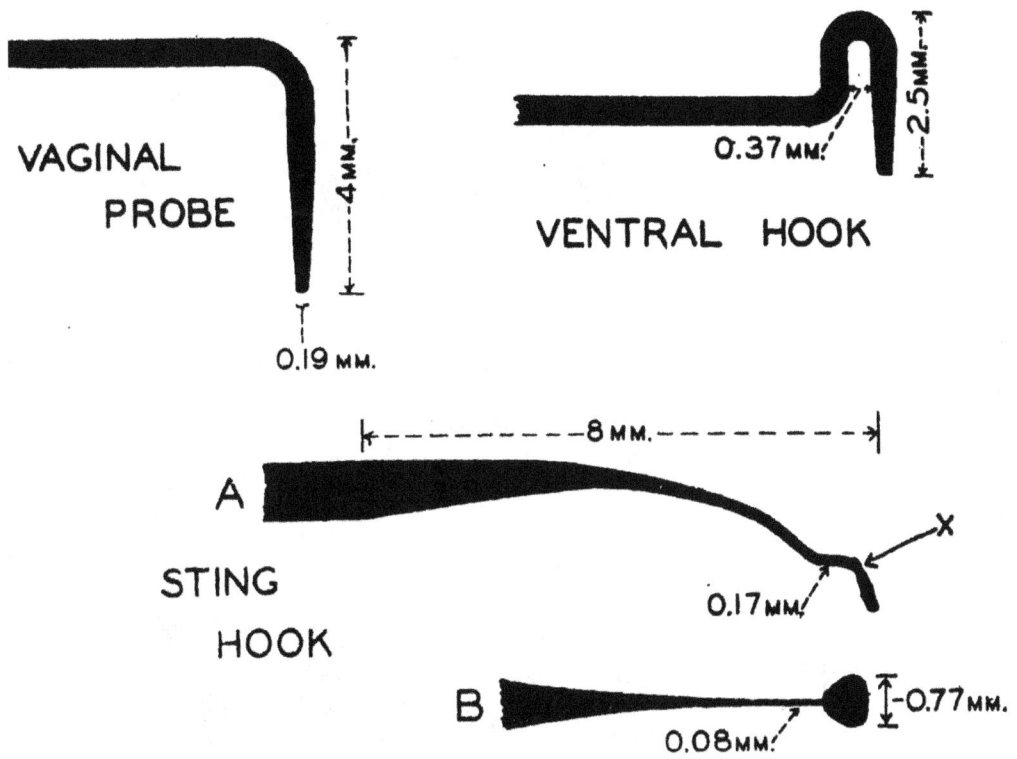

VAGINAL PROBE

4 MM.

0.19 MM.

VENTRAL HOOK

0.37 MM.

2.5 MM.

STING HOOK

A

8 MM.

0.17 MM.

X

B

0.08 MM.

0.77 MM.

Figure 8.—Structural details of vaginal probe, ventral hook (side view), and sting hook with A (side view) and B (top view from the direction indicated by the arrow X). The arrow also marks the point where the end begins to enlarge.

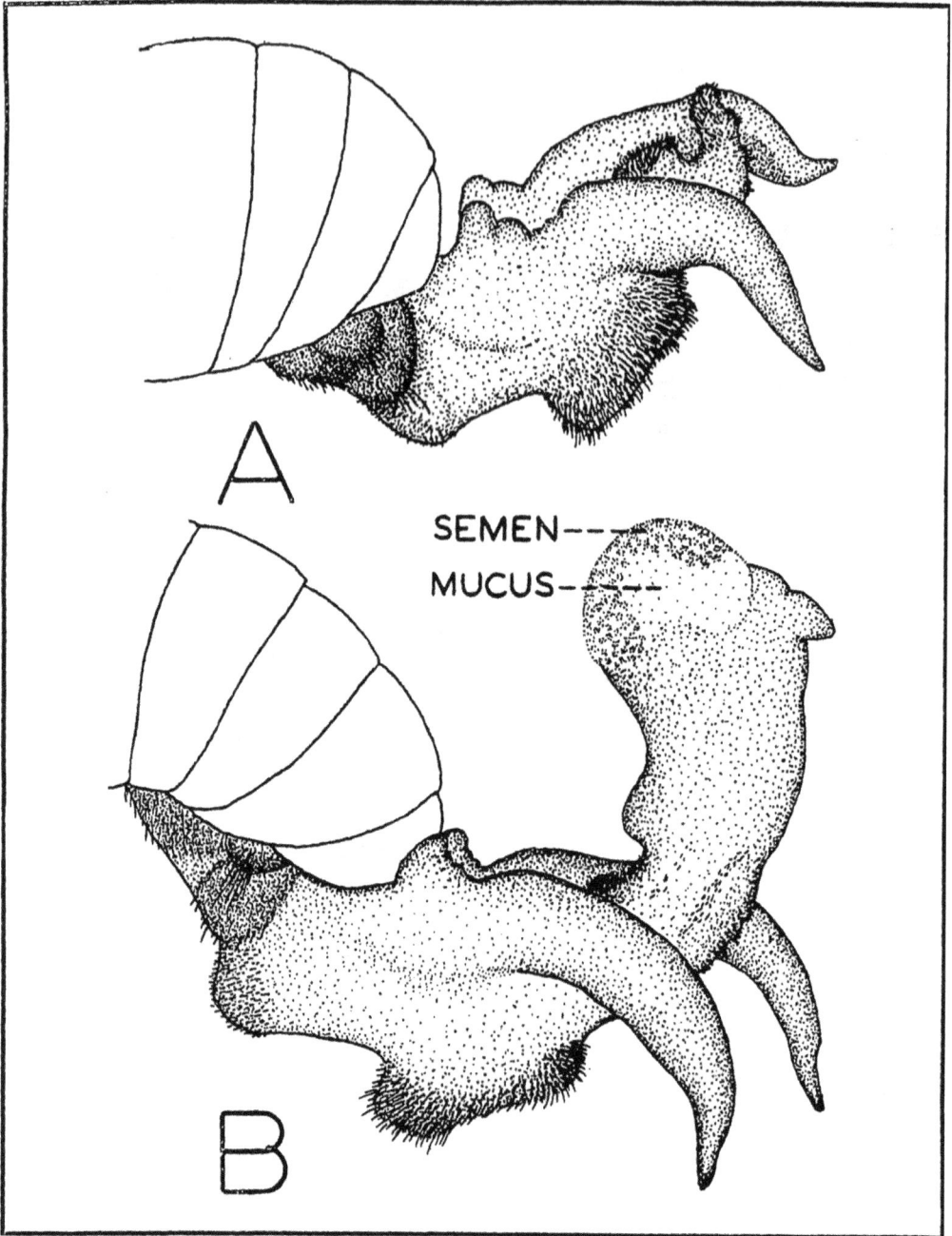

SEMEN---

MUCUS----

Figure 9.—Stages of the eversion of drone's penis: A—partial eversion usually encountered after anesthetization with chloroform; B—a more complete eversion usually obtained by squeezing the abdomen, with semen and mucus exposed.

which is more viscous and will not flow so easily as semen. Mucus is too thick to pass through the end of the syringe easily and will stop the passage of semen. When this happens, the plunger is pushed out until the passage is cleared and then the taking of semen is continued. By moving the syringe about, the mucus can be skimmed of practically all its semen covering. Semen is taken from as many drones as necessary to fill the syringe to the desired point.

As the syringe is filled, it will be noticed that the suction pulls some of the water from around the plunger, thus increasing the amount above the air bubble. Later, as the plunger is pushed out during injection, this water passes back around the plunger. This action will be negligible with a well-made tip. When the plunger is poorly fitted, however, it is sometimes withdrawn as far as it will go before the desired amount of semen has been drawn up. In this case the plunger can be pushed down again while a finger is being held over the end. Such a tip is a time consumer and should be replaced as soon as possible. Some water should remain between the end of the plunger and the air bubble to pass back around the plunger as the semen is injected; otherwise the air bubble, or even some of the semen, may pass around the plunger.

The function of the air bubble is to prevent the mixing of semen and water and to mark the boundary between them so that diluted semen will not be injected. As injection proceeds semen adheres to the side walls and mixes with the water which follows, so that in the absence of an air bubble it is difficult to distinguish between pure and diluted semen. When a series of inseminations is made without the syringe being cleaned, as is possible with the plastic syringe, the air bubble is superfluous.

Injection

As soon as the syringe is filled, the point is moistened to prevent clogging by drying of semen and to lubricate it. The syringe is moved into position over the queen and the microscope pushed forward so that the queen is in the field and the magnification changed to high power. The sting hook is then drawn dorsally until the sting chamber appears as in figure 1. This act stretches the loose membranes so that the vaginal orifice, and often the valvefold, are visible. It also stretches the dorsal wall of the vagina so that the syringe can slide along it into the median oviduct.

With the left hand the probe is inserted into the dorsal part of the vagina and the valvefold pushed ventrally, until the point of the syringe has passed beyond. Then, as the syringe is pushed in farther, the probe is removed. The syringe should be inserted no farther beyond the valvefold than is necessary for satisfactory insemination (about 1 to 1.5 mm.). The plastic tip can be inserted deeper than the glass tip on account of its more gradually tapering point. If it appears that the syringe carries tissue in with it as if caught on the end of the syringe, then the point has not hit the median oviduct and should be withdrawn and reinserted, possibly after some readjustment of the holding hooks.

With the syringe in place the plunger is slowly pushed downward. If the semen moves down the barrel easily and does not leak out around the point, then the syringe is in proper position and the injection can proceed rapidly. If the glass syringe is used, great care must be exercised that the plunger never reaches the cone-shaped point. The plunger of the plastic syringe, on the other hand, can be pushed to the end of the larger bore without danger of breakage.

The syringe is now withdrawn from the queen, and then from its box, the spring being depressed with forceps so that the syringe slips out easily without danger of the point breaking. Removal of the queen from her holder completes the operation.

Cleaning the Syringe

The glass syringe should be cleaned immediately, by alternately drawing in and expelling fresh water until the liquid inside the syringe is relatively clear. When the plunger does not fit closely, a little semen left in the liquid may help to increase suction.

Regardless of the care exercised, a coating gradually accumulates on the inside walls of the syringe, and finally interferes with the passage of semen. This coating can be removed with a piece of wire 0.002 inch in diameter slightly bent at the end. Flakes that are too large to pass through easily can usually be removed by drawing back the plunger slowly so that water passes around and behind them and then pushing out very suddenly so that they will be carried with the stream of water. Several repetitions of this procedure will usually clear the barrel. The glass tip can be cleaned by dipping in a hot solution of an alkali such as sodium hydroxide or common lye, which dissolves the deposits; however, the alkali must be thoroughly rinsed out before the syringe can be used again. When using alkali it is best to withdraw the plunger 15 to 20 mm. and leave the tip full of air, then to draw in a small quantity of the hot alkali. Later the alkali can be forced out and the rinsing done without any contact with the plunger.

The plastic syringe need be cleaned only when it is to be stored or when the plunger becomes too tight. Cleaning is simple. The tip and plunger are unscrewed, and water is drawn in and out with the plunger with such force that usually all obstructions are easily rinsed out.

Sterilizing the Syringe

When a quick change is made from one genetic type of sperm to another, it is necessary to sterilize the syringe. The glass syringe is sterilized by rinsing it thoroughly and then dipping it in boiling water deeply enough to submerge part of the pencil as well as the exposed part of the glass tip, so that the inside end of the tip also becomes heated. If several syringes are available, a fresh one can be employed for each kind of drone used in a single day. The plastic tip is sterilized by quickly drawing in and expelling 95 per cent ethyl alcohol, and then thoroughly rinsing with water immediately, because Lucite is slowly soluble in alcohol.

ESTIMATING THE NUMBER OF SPERMS

One criterion of successful insemination is the number of sperms that reach the spermatheca. A fairly good estimate can be made by the following method:

Items of equipment needed include a counting chamber such as is used to count blood corpuscles, a 50-cc. burette, a medicine-dropper pipette, a small glass dish, a pair of sharp pointed forceps, and a dissecting needle. The pipette should have an inside diameter of about 1 mm. at the tip. For the glass dish an individual saltcellar almost as deep as wide, having a capacity a little over 10 cc., and having a rounded bottom somewhat smaller than the diameter of the rim, has been found to be just the right size and shape.

To dissect out the spermatheca one must tear off the last segment of the abdomen by grasping the last ventral plate with forceps. The spermatheca is usually found imbedded in the tissue inside this removed segment. It is a sphere about 1 mm. in diameter and appears rough and white because of the network of tracheae which covers it completely. When the tracheae are removed, the spermatheca is found to be smooth and transparent in a virgin queen and milky-white to cloudy-cream in mated queens, depending on the degree of insemination.

The spermatheca is placed in the dish and 1 cc. of tap water added from the burette. Then the spermatheca is broken with the sharp-pointed forceps and needle, the sperm teased out, and the empty skin removed. The sperm is dispersed by alternately drawing the water into, and expelling it from, the pipette about twenty times, or until all lumps have disappeared. Then 9 cc. of water is added to make a total of 10 cc. and the sperm again thoroughly dispersed with the pipette. A drop of this mixture is quickly placed in the counting chamber. When the sperm number seems to be small, a dilution to only 5 cc. or less can be used. The sperms are counted under a compound micropscope with a magnification of 60 diameters, and against a dark field, which makes the sperms stand out as white filaments. From the number counted in a certain volume the number in 10 cc. is calculated.

The sperms usually appear as almost headless, slightly curved, filaments about 0.27 mm. long, but they may be coiled or looped into various shapes, such as small circles, spheres, or like the numerals 6 and 8.

It is important that the dispersion be continued no longer than is absolutely necessary and that the drop be placed in the counting chamber quickly before any great amount of settling or adhesion of sperm can take place. It is also important that the pipette be kept clean to prevent lumps of sperm from sticking to its walls. In some localities a physiological salt solution may be more satisfactory than tap water. Distilled water is not recommended.

There is, of course, considerable chance of error in making counts from such a small sample. Nevertheless, this method is certainly more accurate than judging by appearance of the spermatheca and the viscosity of the contents, as has been done by previous investigators. Greater accuracy can be obtained by counting a larger sample. All sperm counts given in this manual were made by diluting individual matings to 5 cc. and other matings to 10 cc. and counting the sperms in 0.8 mm.^{3}.

The number of sperms in the seminal vesicles of drones can be estimated by the same method. A window is carefully cut into the dorsal wall of the abdomen and the seminal vesicles are very gently cut off where they join the muscus glands. If this is not done very carefully, the muscles of the seminal vesicles will contract and some of the sperm will be lost. After being placed in water, the muscles are made to contract by pricking and mashing, and what sperm is not forced out in this way is released by tearing the seminal vesicle to pieces.

THE USE OF CARBON DIOXIDE

Carbon dioxide not only serves as an anesthetic, but also stimulates queens to begin laying (Mackensen 4). Proper treatment with this gas causes virgin as well as inseminated queens to begin laying practically as soon as naturally mated queens, whereas without such treatment only about 20 per cent start earlier than 30 days after emergence.

At least two anesthetizations of 10 minutes duration spaced a day apart are necessary to start egg laying. These may or may not be accompanied by insemination. An anesthetic treatment without insemination is given by placing the caged queen in a convenient container through which carbon dioxide is flowing (fig. 3). If the queen is to begin laying at the normal age (8 to 11 days after emergence), the second treatment must be completed before the seventh day, and preferably before the sixth day, because she begins laying 2 to 6 days after the second treatment. Although treatments given as early as the second and third day are effective, they do not cause laying to start earlier than the normal age.

PROCEDURES FOR VARIOUS TYPES OF MATINGS
AND RESULTS TO BE EXPECTED

Inseminations should be made from the fourth to the tenth day after emergence. They have often been made earlier than this (second and third day), but at times with poor results. At the other extreme, queens can be inseminated at any age if they have not begun laying, but if not made to start soon after the tenth day, they will be balled and mistreated by the worker bees, and the percentage and quality of the laying queens will be reduced.

As much as 10 mm.³ of semen has been given in one operation with success, but because the percentage of sperm that reaches the spermatheca declines as the load increases, it is better to give several small inseminations than a single large one. Except for individual matings, a load of 2.5 to 4.0 mm.³ has been found very satisfactory. Results are also less variable when several inseminations are made than when an equal amount of semen is given in a single insemination. It is best to allow 2 days between inseminations for clearing of semen from the reproductive tract, although often inseminations on successive days have been quite successful. The operation should be performed as rapidly as possible to avoid unnecessary exposure of the sperm.

Individual Matings

Often it is desirable to mate each queen with a single drone. In this case it is important that the maximum possible number of sperms be obtained from the single drone used. Therefore, well-matured, well-nourished drones should be available, and only those used that seem to ejaculate perfectly and to yield a large amount of semen heavy with sperm. The best drones yield nearly 1 mm.³ of semen. Individual matings are usually made only in genetic experiments in which it is imperative that the sperm come from but a single drone. Therefore, if a series of such matings is to be made, the syringe must be sterilized between operations to prevent contamination with sperm previously used. In individual matings the percentage of laying queens is usually high, and most of them will produce some worker offspring. However, so few sperms reach the spermatheca that the supply does not last long, and such matings are only made when absolutely necessary. One additional carbon dioxide treatment must be given to start egg laying.

One Insemination with Sperm from Several Drones

When neither individual mating nor long productive life is desired, several drones from the same source can be used, making one injection consisting of at least 2.5 mm³. of semen. With this procedure it is almost certain that none of the queens will begin laying as partial or complete drone layers, and if kept in nuclei most of them will last a season without becoming drone layers. One additional carbon dioxide treatment is necessary to start egg laying.

Two or More Inseminations

To fill the spermatheca sufficiently to carry a queen through a season in a large colony, two or more inseminations must be made, each consisting of 2.5 mm.³ of semen. An additional carbon dioxide treatment is not necessary. Hundreds of queens mated two or three times have performed as well as naturally mated queens.

A still greater number of sperms can be made to reach the spermatheca by giving three or four inseminations with 2.5 mm.³ of semen. They are given on alternate days beginning on the fourth day or, in the case of four inseminations, they may be started the third day to reduce the likelihood of interference with the beginning of oviposition.

Considerable variation can be expected in the percentage of laying queens obtained. In one group of 95 queens inseminated three times, 83 per cent started laying; however, results as low as 60 per cent can be expected occasionally. In general, the more inseminations made the more chances of injury and consequent loss. Practically all queens that survive to laying age will begin laying.

Table 1 compares the number of sperms in various artificially inseminated and naturally mated queens. These data are taken from several experiments. Note that the coefficient of variation decreases as the number of inseminations is increased, and that it is lower in some of the inseminated queens than in those naturally mated. Note also that the minimum in the group inseminated three times is higher than the minimum in the naturally mated queens, and that the average and maximum in the group inseminated four times are nearly as great as the corresponding figures for the naturally mated queens.

The performance of artificially inseminated queens compares very well with that of naturally mated queens. In 1945 queens inseminated artificially three times were compared with queens of identical parentage mated naturally at an isolated mating station. Surplus honey produced was about the same for the two types of matings, as already reported by Roberts (7). Brood production and brood quality were not significantly different, but survival to the end of the season was somewhat lower in the artificially inseminated group.

TABLE 1.—A comparison between the number of sperm in the spermatheca of naturally mated queens and artificially inseminated queens inseminated as indicated.

TREATMENT.	Number of Queens.	Number of Sperms in Spermatheca (millions).		Coefficient of Variation.
		Average.	Range.	
Artificial insemination:				
Semen from one drone ...	17	0.87	0.22–2.24	51
Semen from many drones (2.5 mm.³)				
Once	11	2.97	1.28–4.41	35
Twice	9	4.11	2.05–5.65	29
Three times	10	4.85	3.71–5.80	16
Four times	11	5.52	4.66–6.79	10
Natural mating	33	5.73	3.34–7.35	18

THE ABSOLUTE CONTROL OF PARENTAGE

The purpose of artificial insemination is the control of parentage, and the virgin queens and drones used are reared from eggs laid by selected breeder queens which are already mated. The virgins are reared from fertilized eggs and inherit from both the breeder queen and the drone with which she mated, whereas the drones develop from unfertilized eggs and inherit only from the breeder queen. These are the desired breeding individuals but occasionally other types of individuals appear in the hive, with which they might be confused. These types are (1) drones and queens reared from unfertilized eggs of laying workers, and (2) queens reared from the unfertilized eggs of the breeder queen. Only the drones are a serious menace to pure mating, but all types will be discussed because they must be considered in the interpretation of genetic experiments.

The number of off-type drones and queens depends largely upon the number of laying workers in the hive which varies considerably with race, season, and hive conditions. Queenlessness for any length of time will cause some workers to start laying, and they may continue to lay after the colony has been made queen right. Laying workers are apparently more common in early spring, when the hive is populated mainly with old, over-wintered bees. They are very common among the Cape bees of South Africa (Jack, 1), but in the bees of the United States and the European races they are relatively rare.

Under conditions where they could be positively identified, 13 off-type drones were found to emerge among about 5,000 drones of the right type reared in a full-sized colony, which is at the rate of 0.26 per cent. Drones have been reared under controlled conditions for a number of seasons, and although the percentage of off-type drones has usually not been determined by actual count, it is estimated not to have exceeded 0.26 per cent. Often none were found among several thousand drones. They can be recognized and avoided if the breeder queen is introduced to a colony of bees of a distinguishable color. For example, if a queen of a yellow strain is introduced to bees of a black strain, her sons and daughters will be yellow and the sons of worker bees will be black.

If a selected breeder queen is supported entirely by her own worker daughters, it is not so important to guard against the off-type individuals, because all descend from the breeder queen and her mate, and therefore represent only the desired germ plasm. Often, however, it is unpractical to wait for a queen to produce her own supporting population.

The other types of undesirable individuals, queens reared from unfertilized eggs of either queen or worker, are called impaternate because they have no male parent. These queens are quite common in some races. Among Cape bees of South Africa laying workers develop readily and produce female offspring in abundance when the hive becomes queenless (Jack, 1). In other races they have been considered to be rare or not to occur at all, but Mackensen (3) has proved their occurrence in three American strains of bees representing the Caucasian and Italian races. He found female progeny in the brood of 21 out of 50 virgin queens tested. Of the larvae grafted from one queen producing a high percentage of female offspring, 0.85 per cent developed into queens. Impaternate females also occur in the related insect " Habrobracon juglandis " Ashm., and Speicher (8) has presented evidence that they develop from diploid eggs which arise from patches of tetraploid tissue in the ovaries.

The frequency with which impaternate daughter queens of laying workers are likely to be encountered in rearing queens by the usual methods has not been determined. If the percentage of impaternate females developing from unfertilized eggs of queens (0.85 per cent) can also be taken as the percentage of laying worker eggs that develop into females, and the rate of occurrence of off-type drones (0.26 per cent) is taken as the percentage of laying worker eggs in the hive, the expected rate of occurrence of queens of this type can be calculated to be 0.0022 per cent, or 1 in 45 thousand. Obviously they are so infrequent that precautions need not be taken to avoid them. If it should be desirable, the method described for off-type drones could be used.

Impaternate queens developing from eggs of the breeder queen inherit only from her. In ordinary breeding work there is no way of recognizing and avoiding them. They probably do not occur among the larvae grafted at all because fertilization would lead to triploidy and probably death, and the larvae ordinarily used for grafting develop from fertilized eggs.

CARE OF QUEENS

To provide the most natural conditions queens are not kept in nursery cages prior to insemination, as recommended by some workers on artificial insemination, but introduced as cells and maintained in nuclei until they begin laying. Excluders are placed over the hive entrances to prevent the loss of queens by mating flights. As soon as possible after emergence, while the queens are still recognizable as newly emerged, one wing is clipped to prevent flight and the thorax is marked with a spot of colour. A lacquer called Libralac mixed with the desired pigment is suitable as a marking fluid. A solution of celluloid in acetone is also a satisfactory vehicle for the pigment.

The queen is taken directly from the nucleus and returned immediately after insemination, while she is still completely motionless from the effect of carbon dioxide. When she is in this condition, the bees are less likely to ball her than if she is active. In warm weather she is dropped into the nucleus, but in cool weather she is left in the cage in which she is transported. The cage is opened and slipped between the top bars of the frames.

REARING AND CARE OF DRONES

It is not always easy to obtain large numbers of drones of the desired parentage. During the spring they can usually be obtained in abundance from any queen, because they are naturally produced at this season, but later in the year it is sometimes almost impossible to obtain any drones at all from some queens. Sometimes, even though the queen will lay in drone comb, the workers refuse to rear larvae to maturity. When a heavy flow is on, the drone comb is filled with fresh nectar so that the queen does not have a chance to lay drone eggs.

Drones are most likely to be obtained out of season if conditions similar to those existing during the swarming season are created. Pollen and sugar syrup can be fed if necessary, and a crowded conditions created either by adding bees and brood or by reducing the size of the hive. When the nectar flow is heavy, empty combs can be provided to help keep the drone comb clear. If drone combs are extracted gently, the thin nectar can be removed without destroying eggs and larvae that might be present in some of the cells.

A sure way to obtain drones is to rear them from drone-laying queens, which can be produced by treating virgin queens with carbon dioxide, as already described. These virgins would, of course, be daughters of the selected breeder queen.

The following routine has been used successfully for a number of years to rear and maintain large numbers of drones of controlled parentage in yellow strains.

A five-frame nucleus is used as a drone-rearing colony. It is made up with three combs of brood from black selected Caucasian stock, a comb of honey, and a drone comb, which is placed in the middle of the nucleus. Extra pollen is provided by sprinkling dry pollen pellets into the combs and spraying with water. The yellow breeder queen is introduced with a push-in cage and released 2 or 3 days later, depending on how well she is accepted. The nucleus is stocked with $3\frac{1}{2}$ pounds of black bees added from a screen cage which covers the top of the nucleus hive. They are forced to go through an excluder, which sifts out drones as they leave the cage. The bees are kept confined for 2 days. Pollen is added occasionally, and the nucleus is sometimes fed very lightly to help stimulate the queen.

As soon as the first drone comb is well filled, another drone comb is substituted for one of the brood combs. This is usually about a week or 10 days after the queen has commenced laying. After another week or 10 days the first drone comb is removed to a drone nursery colony and replaced with a third drone comb. In this way sometimes three or four drone combs can be filled within a month after laying starts.

Special precautions are taken to prevent strange yellow bees, which might develop into laying workers, from drifting into the drone-rearing colony. The colony is established at least 100 yards away from the queen-yard and frequent examinations are made to find and kill any yellow bees that might have drifted in. If other drone-rearing colonies are kept near by, they are removed before yellow bees begin to fly from them.

The drone nursery colony is placed in or very near the queen yard, so that drones from it are conveniently available for insemination. It is kept separated from other bees as much as possible to prevent drifting in of yellow bees. A 1-story 10-frame standard hive is provided with 5 or 6 combs of brood and 4 pounds of bees of black stock added from a screen cage through an excluder, together with some honey and a great excess of pollen. The bees are confined for 2 days. A screen top is placed under the cover, so that ventilation can be provided by lifting the cover slightly when the excluder at the entrance becomes crowded with drones trying to get out. The bees rear their own queen, which remains a virgin because she cannot get out of the hive to mate. Her presence prevents the development of laying workers. More brood is added later to provide a continual supply of young bees.

If the nursery colony is so situated that yellow bees drift in, the drone combs are removed after 24 days, and all other drone brood is killed at 10-day intervals. These precautions are taken to prevent sons of laying workers from maturing, and are unnecessary when the entire worker population is of a body color distinguishable from the drones being nursed by the colony.

All manipulations of the nursery colony are made early in the morning while drones are not normally flying. Often it is necessary to work the colony in a portable screen cage to prevent stray drones from drifting in. After long confinement or when the presence of excluders has kept them out of the hives during the night, drones will often fly in the morning.

The screening of bees for rearing and nursery colonies serves two purposes. It eliminates superfluous black drones which would crowd entrances unnecessarily and also prevents the accidental addition of a queen. For these reasons the procedure has become a matter of routine not only in stocking these colonies but also in stocking nuclei.

At the age of 8 days drones become sexually mature and try to leave the hive. At this age the maximum number of sperms has accumulated in the seminal vesicles, but the drones often do not ejaculate well until they have been trying to get out for a number of days. The feces that accumulate during confinement seem to be an aid rather than a hindrance. Its presence seems to increase the pressure inside the abdomen when the muscles contract, assuring good eversion of the penis and ejaculation. It has been noticed that drones whose flight has not been restricted by confinement to the hive will ejaculate better and in greater numbers after they have been kept in a cage for a day or two with workers, sugar syrup, and pollen. Drones do not live so long when confined as when they are able to fly naturally.

In the nursery colonies some of them die soon after they reach the age of 25 days, and few reach 35 days.

Three important requirements of the drone nursery colony are ample bees, ample pollen, and queenlessness. Drones need the care of worker bees. When kept in cages and provided only with pollen, water, and sugar syrup, they soon die, but when about twice their number of worker bees are added, they live to sexual maturity and contain a good quantity of usable semen. When pollen is omitted drones live for some time, but very few sperms develop. Queenlessness is also necessary when a large number of drones are present; they live longer and mature better in queenless colonies. In 1944 the young drones in two queen-right nursery colonies were noticed massed on the bottom board with not a single one on the combs. After the queens had been removed long enough for the bees to realize their queenlessness, all the drones were found on the combs apparently being well cared for.

SUMMARY

By modification of the equipment and methods of earlier workers on artificial insemination of queen bees, the technique has been improved sufficiently to make its use practical in bee breeding as well as in genetic studies. In this manual the important features of the anatomy of the sex organs, the construction of special equipment, and the insemination procedure are described. The essentials of the method are as follows:

(1) The semen is taken from the everted penis after the drone has been placed in chloroform fumes to induce partial eversion and the abdomen squeezed to continue the eversion until the semen has appeared at the end of the penis.

(2) The semen is deposited in the oviducts in natural mating. To do this it is necessary to push aside a tongue-like projection, from the ventral wall of the reproductive tract, called the valvefold, so that the point of the syringe can reach the median oviduct opening.

(3) The syringe tapers at the end so that its point is small enough to enter the median oviduct, while the main barrel is large enough to have a practical capacity.

(4) At least two inseminations are given at 2-day intervals to approximate the normal number of sperm in the spermatheca.

(5) Carbon dioxide is used as an anesthetic. This gas not only relaxes the queens, but also stimulates them to begin laying. Two anesthetizations of 10 minutes' duration spaced 1 or 2 days apart will cause virgin as well as inseminated queens to begin laying promptly; whereas without this treatment few begin earlier than 30 days after emergence.

Individual matings can be made, but so few sperms (0.87 million) reach the spermatheca that most queens stop laying fertilized eggs within 2 or 3 months. If 2.5 mm.³ of semen, taken from several drones, is given, sufficient sperms (2.97 million) reach the spermatheca to last a season if the queen's laying is restricted by keeping her in a nucleus hive. Two inseminations of this size provide sufficient sperm (4.11 million) to assure fertilized eggs for a season in a full-size colony. With four inseminations of this size almost as many sperms (5.52 million) reach the spermatheca as are found in naturally mated queens (5.73 million).

Sperm numbers are estimated by dispersing the sperms of the spermatheca or of the seminal vesicles of the drone in a given volume of water, counting the number of sperms in a measured sample in a counting-chamber slide, and calculating the number in the total volume.

Queens to be inseminated are introduced as cells and confined to the hive by queen excluders. Soon after emergence the virgins are marked and their wings clipped. They are returned to the nucleus immediately after insemination while they are still completely anesthetized.

When drones are reared from a selected breeder queen, sometimes as high as 0.26 per cent of the drones obtained develop from the unfertilized eggs of laying workers. These off-type drones can be avoided if the breeder queen is first introduced to a colony stocked with worker bees having a body color distinct from that of the breeder queen, so that the drones produced by the worker bees can be recognized and discarded. Virgin queens are also known to develop from unfertilized eggs of laying workers, but are so rare that they need not be considered seriously by the bee breeder.

Drones can usually be produced by creating conditions similar to those existing at swarming time. Crowding of bees, reducing the laying space for the queen, and feeding of sugar syrup and pollen are some of the steps often necessary. A sure way to obtain drones is to produce drone-laying queens by carbon dioxide treatment. Drones in large numbers are best cared for in queenless colonies, confined by queen excluders, with brood, bees, pollen, and honey added as needed.

—— ✳ ——

LITERATURE CITED

(1)   Jack, Rupert W.
        1917. Parthenogenesis amongst the workers of the Cape honey-bee:
              Mr. G. W. Onions' experiments. Roy. Ent. Soc., London, Trans.
              1916: 396–403, illus.

(2)   Laidlaw, H. H., Jr.
        1944. Artificial insemination of the queen bee (" Apis mellifera " L.):
              Morphological basis and results. Jour. Morph. 74: 429–465, illus.

(3)   Mackensen, Otto.
        1943. The occurrence of parthenogenetic females in some strains of
              honey-bees. Jour. Econ. Ent. 36: 465–467.

(4)   ——————
        1947. Effect of carbon dioxide on initial oviposition of artificially
              inseminated and virgin queen bees. Jour. Econ. Ent. 40:
              344–349.

(5)   Nolan, W. J.
        1932. Breeding the honey-bee under controlled conditions. U.S. Dept.
              Agr. Tech. Bul. 326, 49 pp., illus.

(6)   ——————
        1937. Improved apparatus for inseminating queen bees by the Watson
              method. Jour. Econ. Ent. 30: 700–705, illus.

(7)   Roberts, W. C.
        1946. The performance of the queen bee. Amer. Bee Jour. 86: 185–186,
              211, illus.

(8)   Speicher, Kathryn G., and B. R. Speicher.
        1938. Diploids from unfertilized eggs in " Habrobracon." Biol. Bul.
              74: 247–252, illus.

(9)   Watson, Lloyd R.
        1927. Controlled mating of queen bees. 50 pp., illus. Hamilton, Ill.

(10)   ——————
        1929. New contributions to the technique of instrumental insemination
              of queen bees. Jour. Econ. Ent. 22: 944–954, illus.